FROM HEART TO MOUTH

The amazing nutrient coenzyme Q-10 has been shown to be helpful in such disparate conditions as life-threatening cardiomyopathy and periodontal disease. Because of its antioxidant effect and its role in the production of cellular energy, it is also often effective in managing diabetes and obesity, in detoxification and longevity, and in sustaining the immune system. With virtually no side effects reported in international studies, and with many verified remarkable health benefits, coenzyme Q-10 should be investigated by all concerned with maintaining or regaining good health.

ABOUT THE AUTHOR

William H. Lee, R.Ph., Ph.D. practiced pharmacy, had his doctorate in nutrition and a Master Herbalist's degree. He wrote for many popular, professional and trade magazines such as *Vegetarian Times* and *Modern Maturity*, was the nutrition columnist for *American Druggist* magazine and lectured frequently to both the layperson and professionals. His major books included *The Book of Raw Fruits and Vegetable Juices*, *Concentrated Healing Foods* and *The Question and Answer Book of Vitamins*.

Coenzyme Q-10

Is it our new fountain of youth?

William H. Lee, R.Ph., Ph.D.

Keats Publishing, Inc.　　New Canaan, Connecticut

Coenzyme Q-10 is not intended as medical advice. Its intention is solely informational and educational. Please consult a medical or health professional should the need for one be indicated.

Keats Good Health Guides™ are published by
Keats Publishing, Inc.
27 Pine Street (Box 876)
New Canaan, Connecticut 06840-0876

Contents

Acknowledgments

The author acknowledges that material received from the following companies enabled this book to be completed.

Solgar Co., Inc.
Lynbrook, New York 11563

Twin Laboratories, Inc.
Ronkonkoma, New York 11779

Cardiovascular Research, Ltd.
Concord, CA 94518

Phoenix Laboratories, Inc.
Hicksville, New York 11802

The Life Extension Foundation
Hollywood, Florida 33020

The body is a collection of systems working together for the good of the whole. The body cannot function at its best unless all systems are performing at peak efficiency. We usually think of this collection in terms of the individual systems, such as the digestive system, the respiratory system, the reproductive system, and so forth. Such a perception is adequate for most purposes but, unfortunately, it does not go far enough for the purposes of this book.

Each system has an effect on other systems. Mental stress can cause digestive problems, sexual problems, and headaches. Eating the wrong foods can cause lethargy, lack of concentration, and loss of energy. Constipation can cause nausea, dizziness, and lack of appetite. What bothers any one system ends up disrupting all of the other systems in one way or another.

When we think of systems, we usually think of them as wholes rather than their components. We should think of a system as a collection of individual cells that, together, make up the system. Each cell is a miniature body. It carries on all of the functions of the body including ingestion, digestion, waste removal, and reproduction. It is the individual cell's health that is vitally important to the total health of the body. If the individual cell is kept supplied with adequate nutrition and if it functions as it should, then the system functions, and the body functions. But, should the individual cell falter, it is the beginning of problems for the entire body structure and, perhaps, the disease we call aging!

All systems, internal or external, run on energy. Food is the important source of energy to the body and to the individual cell. Each cell has a miniature engine within it that converts the nutrients it receives into the energy it must have to carry on its activities. If a cell does not receive nutrients, it will not be able to carry on its functions and to reproduce itself as a perfect cell. The production of imperfect cells can be called aging, and is detected by wrinkles, sagging skin, loss of hair, loss of memory, and other consequences. A starved cell will not perform as a perfect part of the whole body. Nutritional deficiency will affect muscle status, circulation, cardiovascular health, blood pressure, and the immune system.

Because coenzyme Q-10 is found in every cell in the body, it is the key to the process that produces 95 percent of cellular energy.

Without coenzyme Q-10, we wouldn't have enough energy to stay alive! Coenzyme Q-10 may be the ultimate antidote to aging, the life-force your body produces to stay alive and healthy . . . and it can be taken as a nutritional supplement!

Coenzyme Q is also known as ubiquinone. The name was formed from the word *ubiquitous* and the coenzyme *quinone*, because coenzyme Q is found in virtually every cell in the body.

Ubiquinone is a naturally occurring substance with a molecular structure that is similar to vitamin K. It is found in humans, animals, and plants. The form naturally present in plants is known as plastaquinone. Animals and humans have a variety of molecular formulations ranging from coenzyme Q-6 to coenzyme Q-10. The difference in the numbered designations refers to the number of isoprene units in the molecular chain. Coenzyme 6 to coenzyme 10 are found in animals, while only coenzyme Q-10 is found in humans. Although coenzyme Q-10 is the form utilized by the body for its energy function, the animal forms can be raised to the Q-10 position when ingested as part of the diet.

The richest source of the coenzyme for supplemental purposes is beef heart. Although initial investigations were carried out using this source, the expense of extracting the coenzyme made general use prohibitive. The Japanese later discovered a fermentation process and have mass-produced it at affordable levels.

Although this substance shows remarkable promise and safety in its ability to normalize many critical body situations such as cardiovascular disease, hypertension, and periodontal disease, it has not been approved by the Food and Drug Administration as anything but a food supplement. Karl Folkers, biomedical researcher at the University of Texas at Austin, holds the Food and Drug Administration permit to test the substance as a treatment for heart problems.

One of the basic precepts of nutritional healing is illustrated by coenzyme Q-10. If the enzyme is low or deficient in the body, coenzyme Q-10 therapy is likely to be rewarding. If the level of coenzyme Q-10 is normal, the addition of supplemental coenzyme Q-10 will usually have little or no effect.

ENZYMES AND COENZYMES

Enzymes are protein substances found in plants, animals, humans, and all living things. They are necessary for the building and rebuilding of tissues and cells. Enzymes are catalysts that influence all life systems from our heads to our toes. They are produced by living cells but are capable of acting independently. They are complex proteins that can induce chemical changes in other substances without being changed themselves. Enzymes are specific in their action; they will act only on a certain substance or a group of closely related substances and no others.

Enzymes consist of at least two parts: the protein portion and the cofactor portion. The specific amino acids that compose the protein portion of the enzyme are determined by the genetic code. Either mineral ions (such as calcium, magnesium, and zinc) or vitamins, or both in some instances, make up the cofactor portion of the complete enzyme. The vitamin portion is usually called the coenzyme.

Most people know a little about the workings of a car engine. To help us understand the way energy is used in the body, it may be useful to use the analogy of the automobile. The individual cell, of course, is far more complex than the gasoline engine in a car, but they are analogous.

In an automobile engine, the proper mixture of gasoline with oxygen ignites to provide the necessary energy to drive the pistons. Various gears and linkages harness this energy to turn the wheels. Within this framework energy can be viewed as the capacity or ability to do work. Increasing or decreasing the energy supply either speeds up or slows down the engine. Similarly, the human body must continuously be supplied with its own form of energy to perform its many complex operations. Aside from the energy needed for work performed by the muscle system, there is a considerable demand for energy by other forms of biologic work. This includes the energy for digestion, absorption, and assimilation of the food nutrients. It includes, also, energy for the functioning of various glands that secrete special hormones, for the establishment of the proper electrochemical gradients along the cell membrane to permit transmission of brain signals through the nerves to the muscles, and for the building of new chemical compounds such as protein. *All of this energy begins in the individual cell.*

ATP, the Engine's Fuel. The cell's engine is called the *mitochondria*. The enzyme that makes it all work is succinate dehydrogenase-co-Q-10 reductase. The cells do not use the nutrients consumed in the diet for their immediate supply of energy. Instead, they prepare an energy-rich compound called *adenosine triphosphate*, or simply ATP.

ATP is the "fuel" used for *all* the energy-requiring processes within the cell. In turn, the energy in food is extracted to build more ATP. The potential energy stored in the ATP molecule represents chemical energy made in the cell as it is needed.

Molecules are composed of atoms held together by bonds. It is the breaking of the ATP molecule's bonds that releases energy. ATP consists of one molecule of adenine and ribose called *adenosine*, combined with three phosphates and oxygen atoms. A considerable amount of energy is stored in the ATP molecule at the bonds that link the two outermost phosphate groups with the remainder of the molecule. When the outermost bond is broken, it releases an amount of energy equivalent to approximately 7,000 calories.

$$\text{ADENOSINE} - \text{O} - \underset{\underset{\text{OH}}{|}}{\overset{\overset{\text{O}}{\|}}{\text{P}}} - \text{O} - \underset{\underset{\text{OH}}{|}}{\overset{\overset{\text{O}}{\|}}{\text{P}}} - \text{O} - \underset{\underset{\text{OH}}{|}}{\overset{\overset{\text{O}}{\|}}{\text{P}}} - \text{OH}$$

This equation is the chemical reason for 95% of the energy required for the operation of the body.

Although ATP serves as the energy current for *all* cells, its quantity is limited. In fact, only about three ounces of ATP are stored in the body at any one time! This would provide only enough energy to sustain strenuous activity, such as running as fast as you can, for 5 to 8 seconds. Therefore, ATP must be constantly synthesized to provide a continuous supply of energy. If it were not constantly produced, our "fuel tanks" would read "empty" and all movement would cease. The foods we eat and store in ready access within the body provide the basic raw material to change into ATP with the help of coenzyme Q-10.

The body extracts the potential energy stored within the

structure of carbohydrate, fat, and protein molecules consumed in the diet or stored in the body. This energy is harnessed for one major purpose, to combine adenosine and phosphate to form the energy-rich compound ATP.

Coenzyme Q-10. Ubiquinone, another name for coenzyme Q-10, was formed from the word *ubiquitous* because the enzyme was found in all of the cells of the body. It is a naturally occurring molecule that resembles the chemical structure of vitamin K in molecular appearance. It is the cofactor in the electron transport chain, the biochemical pathway in cellular respiration from which ATP and most of the body's energy are derived.

Because the body must have available energy to carry on the simplest operation, for example breathing in oxygen and breathing out carbon dioxide, coenzyme Q-10 is considered essential for the health of all the body cells, tissues, and organs.

The metabolic pathways in which coenzyme Q-10 participates have been termed "bioenergetics" by Karl Folkers. Folkers was a pioneer researcher in the synthesis of coenzyme Q-10, since its initial source, from beef hearts, made the raw material quite expensive. The Japanese have used a fermentation process to produce coenzyme Q-10 for the mass market for several years. This has enabled six million Japanese to use this unique supplement on a daily basis at a low cost. Although the body can produce this substance, deficiencies have been reported in a wide range of clinical conditions. We will go into the individual diseases associated with coenzyme Q-10 deficiency a bit later in this booklet.

Animal studies have shown that the decline in coenzyme Q-10 levels that occur with age may be partly responsible for age-related deterioration of the immune system. In one animal study, E.Z. Bliznakov (1978) found that coenzyme Q-10 declined by 80 percent in the course of normal aging. A decline of this magnitude in a human being would be fatal, but deficiencies approaching this have been observed in aged humans and are associated with grave heart disease.*

Human cells contain coenzyme Q-10, while animal cells have coenzyme Q-6 to Q-10. Plants, algae, and the photosynthetic bacteria contain a substance that is similar to the enzyme. The plant substances are called plastaquinones. Although the animal structure can be raised from coenzyme Q-6 to coenzyme Q-10 in the body, there is some question whether plastaquinones

*References to the published reports on this substance are given in the Bibliography at the end of this booklet.

could act as a supplement if coenzyme Q-10 is required. Synthesis of the enzyme from plant sources through chemical modification is, however, entirely possible.

Coenzyme Q-10 supplements. A need for supplemental Q-10 could arise for several reasons:

1. Impaired coenzyme Q-10 synthesis due to nutritional deficiencies
2. Genetic or acquired defect in coenzyme Q-10 synthesis
3. Increased tissue needs resulting from a particular medical condition

Because of its role in energy production, a deficiency of the enzyme could cause or aggravate many medical conditions.

If taken orally, coenzyme Q-10 can be taken up and utilized by the body. Because coenzyme Q-10 plays such an important role in energy production and can be administered orally, it is possible to correct a deficiency of the enzyme and the metabolic associated consequences by supplementing with it.

The early research done with coenzyme Q-10 used the Q-7 form, which the body converted to the Q-10 form. Although the body is capable of converting Q-7 into the natural form, coenzyme Q-10 is now commercially available from a number of companies.

Deficiency Documentation. Coenzyme Q-10 participates in the Krebs (citric acid) cycle enzyme system known as succinate dehydrogenase-CoQ10 reductase. In order to detect a deficiency in this enzyme, an assay of its activity is performed. If the enzyme is fully saturated with coenzyme Q-10, then supplementation will not increase the activity. If, on the other hand, tissue levels are shown to be low, the use of supplemental coenzyme Q-10 will increase the activity appreciably.

COENZYME Q-10 IN CLINICAL MEDICINE

Coenzyme Q-10 is present in all body cells. Within the cells it is found in the cytosol (soluble cell fraction) and in the mitochondria (a cellular organelle). The major portion of cellular coenzyme Q-10 is present in the mitochondria as part of the electron transport system. It is in this system that oxidative phosphorylation, a critical link to life itself, and the rate of oxidation of nutrients are regulated. Thus, the heart and the liver, which are both central to this process, contain the largest number of mitochondria per cell and the greatest amount of coenzyme Q-10.

Cardiovascular Disease. In the heart, cellular mitochondria provide energy for the intake of nutrients and for the constant pumping action. The heart muscle utilizes triglycerides prepared by the liver as fuel to generate its energy; thus the heart is entirely dependent on mitochondrial phosphorylation to generate the energy needed for nonstop action.

The action of promoting better functioning of the myocardial tissue is one component of an overall treatment program for cardiovascular disease. Frequently, however, it is overlooked by the profession. The pumping function can be impaired by degenerative lesions. These lesions can be found in most types of cardiovascular problems such as hypertension, atherosclerosis, valvular heart disease, and primary cardiomyopathy.

It is possible that the lesions result from repeated insults to the cardiac tissue from a variety of reasons. They can include ischemic events, inflammation, the release of catecholamines in greater than normal amounts due to stress (emotional or physical), as well as other factors.

If optimum nutrition is supplied at the cellular level, which means diet, vitamins and minerals, as well as coenzyme Q-10, it appears that degeneration may be delayed or forestalled and that the mechanical action of the heart may be improved.

Animal studies and human tests have clearly shown the results of the supplementation with coenzyme Q-10. In animals, coenzyme Q-10 reduced the infarct size resulting from acute coronary occlusion and protected the myocardium against experimentally induced cardiomyopathy and myocarditis.

A deficiency of coenzyme Q-10 is common in cardiac patients. When it was looked for, myocardial biopsies done on patients with various cardiac diseases showed that there was a deficiency of the enzyme in 50 to 75 percent of the patients studied.

Because the heart is so metabolically active and needs the constant supply of usable fuel for its constant contraction and pumping action, it may be unusually susceptible to the effects of coenzyme Q-10 deficiency. Conversely, coenzyme Q-10 has shown to be a supplement of great promise in the treatment of heart disease.

Angina Pectoris. According to *Taber's Cyclopedic Medical Dictionary*, angina pectoris causes severe pain and feeling of pressure in the region of the heart. It is accompanied with great anxiety, fear of approaching death, sweating, and ashen or livid face. Attacks may be brief or last for a considerable period. The prognosis may be grave. Attacks may be intermittent, and with proper rest and care, recovery is possible.

A small study, at least in the number of patients involved if not in importance, was done on twelve patients with stable angina pectoris (Kamikawa, 1985). They were given 150 milligrams of coenzyme Q-10 daily for four weeks. The patients being given the supplement were compared to a second group receiving a medication that looked like coenzyme Q-10 but was really only milk sugar. Neither the patients nor the doctors knew who was receiving what. At the end of the test, results were compared.

Compared to the placebo patients, the patients receiving the real supplement had reduced the frequency of anginal episodes by 53 percent. There was also a significant increase in treadmill exercise tolerance (time to onset of chest pain and time to the development of ST-segment depression) during the treatment.

Since there have been no side reactions to the use of coenzyme Q-10 in the dosages prescribed, the results suggest that coenzyme Q-10 might be a safe and effective treatment for angina pectoris under the supervision of a competent health practitioner.

Congestive Heart Failure. Several studies were run concerning the use of coenzyme Q-10 and congestive heart failure (Ishiyama, 1976).

In one study, seventeen patients suffering from mild congestive heart failure (CHF) were given thirty milligrams of coenzyme Q-10 daily. After four weeks results were tabulated. All patients improved and nine of the patients no longer showed any symptoms of the disease. In other words, 53 percent of the patients treated were asymptomatic in four weeks.

Another study included twenty patients with congestive heart failure due either to ischemic (local or temporary deficiency of the blood supply due to obstruction of the circulation to the heart) or hypertensive heart disease. Treatment included thirty milligrams of coenzyme Q-10 every day for one to two months. Fifty-five percent of the patients reported subjective improvement. Fifty percent showed a decrease in New York Heart Association classification. Thirty percent showed a "remarkable" decrease in chest congestion as proven by chest X-rays. The milder the disease, the greater the improvement, although those patients with a more severe problem showed improvement as well.

The patients who had reported subjective improvement were given a series of tests to bear out their reported findings. The researchers tested stroke volume, cardiac output, cardiac index and ejection fraction. Test results showed the improvement in cardiac function consistent with the patients' reports.

Results were consistent with a positive inotropic effect of coenzyme Q-10, although the effect was not as powerful as that of the cardiac drug digitalis. In addition, coenzyme Q-10 prevented the negative effect of beta-blocker therapy without reducing the beneficial effects of the beta-blockers on myocardial oxygen consumption.

Digitalis has been used in severe cases of congestive heart failure, but the chance of digitalis toxicity at the dose necessary to attempt to correct the problem is always present. There is a possibility that a combination of digitalis and coenzyme Q-10 might reduce the needed dosage of digitalis and the accompanying risk.

The remarkable safety of coenzyme Q-10 and the almost total lack of toxicity at the dosages prescribed appear to suggest that it might possibly replace conventional therapy and become the treatment of choice for mild congestive heart failure. Coenzyme Q-10 might also be an adjunctive therapeutic agent to be used along with beta-blockers to prevent the impairment of cardiac functions that sometimes appear during this therapy.

Since coenzyme Q-10 is a natural substance produced within the body, and since the body also responds to it as a supplement, and it appears to be effective in treating mild cases of congestive heart failure by increasing the intrinsic strength of the heart muscle, it would appear to be a subject for very close scrutiny by the medical community. However, at this time it is sold only as a nutritional supplement in the United States, to maintain health.

Cardiomyopathy. Cardiomyopathy is a term which usually refers to a disease of the heart muscles of obscure etiology. The diagnosis of cardiomyopathy is difficult, but doctors believe this disease is killing thousands of patients yearly. The substance coenzyme Q-10, still not accepted by the FDA, offers the promise of being the first substance effective for the disease.

According to an article in the *Miami Herald* for December 19,

1985, Earl Weed of Temple, Texas, was so sick with a diagnosed case of cardiomyopathy that it was all he could do to sit up. Weed began taking treatments of synthetic coenzyme Q-10, a lab copy of a natural substance needed by the heart to convert food and oxygen into life-giving energy. The results were remarkable, the 61-year-old man recalled. "I've been painting my house inside and out. If I can do that, I can do most everything."

Deficiency of coenzyme Q-10 has been uncovered in the myocardial tissue and in the blood of patients suffering from severe cardiomyopathy. Where there was evidence of a deficiency, supplementation of the enzyme was begun on patients with diagnosed cardiomyopathy. Oral supplementation for two to eight months increased the level of the enzyme in the myocardial tissue in the patients. In some, the increase was greater than in others. In a double-blind study with the use of 100 milligrams of coenzyme Q-10 daily for twelve weeks, it was determined that shortness of breath and increased cardiac muscle strength showed the benefits of supplementation. These shown improvements lasted for as long as three years in patients treated continuously. In contrast, when the use of the supplement was discontinued, the cardiac function deteriorated.

There are no firm statistics on deaths due to cardiomyopathy because of the difficulty in diagnosis, but Dr. Eugene Morkin, professor of medicine at the University of Arizona Health Science Center, where almost 100 heart transplant operations have been performed, said that cardiomyopathy was a major problem for about one third of the patients. He also said that those suffering from the disease do not respond well to conventional therapy.

Dr. Per Langsjoen of Scott & White Memorial Hospital in Tempe, Arizona, when reporting on his research done in Tokyo, Japan, was supportive of coenzyme Q-10 therapy. He said that cardiomyopathy patients steadily worsening and expected to die within two years under conventional therapy generally showed an extraordinary clinical improvement when given coenzyme Q-10, indicating that the supplemental therapy might extend their lives (Judy, 1984).

In an open trial, 34 patients with severe congestive cardiomyopathy were given 100 milligrams of coenzyme Q-10 daily. Eighty-two percent of the patients improved with the supplement. The two-year survival rate increased to 62 percent compared to less than 25 percent for a similar group of patients treated by conventional methods but without added coenzyme Q-10.

In Japan, coenzyme Q-10 is used to treat several cardiac diseases. Eisai Co. Ltd., of Tokyo, has been marketing it under the trade name Neuquinon since 1974. Neuquinon is also sold in Korea, Taiwan, and Italy.

Hyperthyroid Heart Failure. Overstimulation of the thyroid gland and excess thyroxin secretion can cause huge problems to the body. The symptoms include exophthalmia (bulging of the eyes), weight loss, heat intolerance, excessive nervousness, irritability, elevated heart rate, elevated blood pressure, and muscle weakness.

Serum coenzyme Q-10 levels appear to be significantly lower than normal levels in patients with hyperthyroidism. Because congestive heart failure may occur as a result of the thyroid condition or as a result of the decreased amount of the enzyme, 120 milligrams of coenzyme Q-10 daily were given for one week to twelve hyperthyroid patients. The patients' hearts, already stimulated by the condition far past the normal action, responded with augmented performance (Suzuki, 1984).

It is possible that coenzyme Q-10 has a therapeutic value for congestive heart failure induce by thyrotoxicosis. This area is one which should be investigated further by qualified researchers. A recent book by Stephen E. Langer, M.D., *Solved: The Riddle of Illness*, Keats Publishing, New Canaan, Conn., attributes many of the health problems suffered by people to the thyroid gland.

Mitral Valve Prolapse. A cardiac evaluation was made of 194 children with symptomatic mitral valve prolapse using the standard isometric hand grip test (Oda, 1984). All of the tested patients showed an abnormal response to hand grip previous to supplementation.

Eight of the children were given two milligrams per kilogram of body weight every day for eight weeks while a control group of eight children were given placebo tablets of milk sugar that physically resembled the tablets of coenzyme Q-10. At the end of the eighth week, all of the children were tested again. The hand grip test became normal for seven of the eight children who received the coenzyme Q-10, but none of the children who had received the placebo tablet showed any improvement.

Relapse to the former condition was frequently noted in those patients who discontinued using the supplement within one year to 17 months, but rarely occurred in those patients who continued to use the coenzyme Q-10 for 18 months or longer.

Hypertension. Systolic pressures of 140 to 150 mm Hg. and diastolic pressures of 90 to 100 mm Hg. are generally regarded as the upper limits of normal to slightly high blood pressure. Sustained elevation of systolic pressure, diastolic pressure, or both, above these limits is termed hypertension.

If a cause of the hypertension can be determined, the hypertensive state is called secondary hypertension. That is, it occurs secondary to some other demonstrable disorder. If no specific cause for the hypertension can be discerned, the hypertension is designated as essential or primary hypertension.

Among the causes of secondary systolic hypertension are increased cardiac output, and rigidity of the walls of the aorta and main arteries (arteriosclerosis).

Diastolic hypertension appears to be particularly dangerous and can result in vascular damage that may affect the operation of the organs that the affected vessels serve. Vessels serving the kidneys, liver, pancreas, brain, and retina appear to be particularly prone to damage.

When 59 patients with hypertension were tested for the presence of coenzyme Q-10, 39 percent showed a deficiency. As a control, 65 people with normal pressure were also tested for coenzyme Q-10. Of this group, only six percent showed a deficiency (Yamagami, 1977).

Twenty-five patients suffering from essential hypertension were given supplemental coenzyme Q-10, 60 milligrams a day for eight weeks. The results showed a highly significant decrease in blood pressure in the group as a whole. The results also showed that 54 of the test group had a mean blood pressure drop greater than ten percent less than the pressure at the start of the test (Yamagami, 1974).

Thus, coenzyme Q-10 is not a typical antihypertensive drug but a natural substance that appears to correct some metabolic abnormality, which, in turn, has a favorable influence on blood pressure.

The effect of the supplement is not instantaneous. Results are not usually seen until after therapy has been continued for anywhere from four to twelve weeks. This delay in perceptible results is consistent with the gradual buildup in enzyme activity that has appeared in other coenzyme Q-10 therapy.

In animal studies of experimental hypertension, it was found that induced hypertension led to a deficiency of coenzyme Q-10, which was then corrected by addition of the supplement. Whether coenzyme Q-10 deficiency is a cause or an effect of hypertension, correction of the deficiency may improve the blood pressure in selected cases.

Coenzyme Q-10 has reduced aldosterone secretion in dogs and inhibited the sodium-retaining effect of aldosterone and angitensis in rats. Other animal tests involving spontaneously hypertensive rats and experimentally hypertensive dogs have also shown response to oral coenzyme Q-10.

COENZYME Q-10 AND LONGEVITY

According to nutritional science, we should live to the ripe old age of 125 or more. We, all of us, are being cheated out of many enjoyable and productive years because of degenerative diseases common to aging.

Who wants to grow old the way that degeneration has made old age in the commonest sense? Who wants the sagging skin, the wrinkles, the bulges of fat that appear as if by magic one day and refuse to leave us?

Who wants a menu restricted to the blandest of foods and a life dependent on the vicinity of the nearest bathroom?

Failing memory, indigestion, constipation or diarrhea on a regular basis—who wants these? Who wants just enough energy to get us through the day. And sex—did it leave with the failing memory? Tooth troubles, gum trouble, bone troubles, . . . trouble everywhere are the too-common companions of aging.

We can assume that aging is the way nature limits the number of lives on earth to make room for new generations, and that it is impossible to leave this earth alive. But why be cheated out of up to fifty years of life that is available to us according to the laws of nature?

Longevity and Nutrition. For a longer life, nutritional intervention can be an answer. The biogenic potential for a longer life is a possibility for those who decide to take matters into their own hands and investigate the body and its systems: energy, digestion, assimilation, and elimination

The average American diet will do little to extend life. If it did, there wouldn't be millions of Americans suffering from cardiovascular disease, diabetes, cancer, hypertension, and a host of other degenerative ailments. About two-thirds of our people are suffering from chronic malnutrition, leading to obesity and to the killer diseases from failing livers and failing kidneys.

It should be obvious that changing one's diet will contribute to a longer life. Switching over to complex carbohydrates, raw fruits, raw or lightly steamed vegetables, fish and fowl will help. Eliminating canned, processed, and refined foods, and eating foods in season will also improve the body systems. But, there are also "uncommon" supplementary suggestions which can help to ward off the insults the body has to endure.

As you have read, this book has to do with coenzyme Q-10 and its involvement with the generation of essential energy. The heart and the liver contain the largest number of mitochondria (fuel cells) per tissue concentration, therefore, the greatest amount of coenzyme Q-10 and the greatest need for the enzyme.

The mitochondria contain a large number of enzymes organized and grouped together according to their function, e.g., electron transport enzymes, citric acid cycle enzymes and fatty acid alteration enzymes.

These enzyme systems require coenzymes, which, in many cases, are derived from vitamins. In particular, the B-complex family of vitamins such as vitamin B3 (niacin) and vitamin B2 (riboflavin). Niacin is involved in the production of nicotinic acid-nicotinamine adeninedenucleotide (NAD), and riboflavin in riboflavin-flavineodenine dinucleotide (FAD).

The important cofactor in the electron transport chain and the mitochondria is coenzyme Q-10. It plays the critical role in the pumping of protons across the mitochondrial membrane. As we age, the amount of coenzyme Q-10 in the body declines.

In humans, coenzyme Q-10 serves the following purposes that may be connected to the aging process:

1. Increases energy and exercise tolerance. Most aging people claim they do not have the energy to exercise or even to do more moderate amounts of walking. This may be the result of a deficiency of the enzyme or may be a sedentary habit.
2. Corrects age-related declines in the immune system which can leave the body easy prey to bacterial and viral infection. Mouse experiments have shown that coenzyme Q-10 is able

to partially correct declines in the immune system of mice related to age. It is possible that coenzyme Q-10 is a significant immunologic stimulant.

3. Has considerable healing effect on age-related periodontal disease. When people can keep their teeth longer, they can eat better and keep their nutrition at peak level. (More will be said about coenzyme Q-10 and periodontal disease later in this booklet.)

4. Defuses peroxides from within and without the body. The antioxidant action of certain nutrients have been shown to exert an important influence on longevity. Free radicals, highly reactive particles, damage the cells and the cell nucleus. The damaged cell cannot reproduce an undamaged cell because the blueprint for cell-building has been harmed. As a result an inefficient cell is formed with the potential for building another damaged cell, and so on. Antioxidant nutrients such as vitamin E react with the free radicals to render them harmless. Coenzyme Q-10 has a chemical structure that is similar to that of vitamin E, which may account for its potent antioxidant ability. Coenzyme Q-10 is able to inhibit lipid peroxidation in the membrane of the mitochondria, peroxidation which would attack the cell membrane and severely limit its energy-making potential.

It is strange but true that the very process of producing energy also generates free radicals. Coenzyme Q-10, when it is present in sufficient quantities, is in a perfect position to squelch these overactive molecules as soon as they are formed.

Coenzyme Q-10 and Detoxification. In addition to the direct anti-aging effects shown by this enzyme, it also appears that it is able to act against the possible toxic side effects of some prescription drugs used to treat older people for common illnesses of aging. (More will be said about this later in connection with adriamycin.)

One of the least discussed and most important of all of the body systems for promoting long life and health is the liver. The liver is responsible for nutrient assimilation and storage as well as detoxifying the body system and eliminating poisons that might accumulate in the body. The liver is the largest solid organ in the body and weighs about four pounds. It is a chemical plant that can modify almost any chemical structure.

A powerful detoxifying organ, it can break down a variety of toxic molecules, rendering them harmless. It is a storage organ and a blood reservoir. It stores vitamins A and D, digested carbohydrates, and glycogen, which is released to sustain blood sugar levels. The liver manufactures enzymes, cholesterol, proteins, and blood coagulation factors.

One of the prime functions of the liver is to produce bile which promotes efficient digestion of fats. It synthesizes amino acids used in building tissues, it breaks up proteins into sugar and fat when they are needed as such, and it produces urea, and it is closely connected with normal calcium metabolism.

Studies have shown that the aging liver is often operating at less than peak efficiency. Although the liver employs several pathways for energy generation, mitochondrial oxidative phosphorylation is the major pathway for generating energy. As we have read throughout this booklet, this pathway requires quantities of coenzyme Q-10.

Life extension requires many nutrients, among them the essential mineral selenium. Selenium is a potent anticancer agent and an antioxidant. There is some evidence that the use of selenium as a supplement also elevates the coenzyme Q-10 content in the tissues of laboratory rats. Magnesium, another necessary mineral, also appears to stimulate the production of the enzyme within the body.

It is remarkable that many diverse dietary and hormonal alterations that can promote longevity also elevate coenzyme Q-10 levels.

Nevertheless coenzyme Q-10 levels are depressed by interventions that adversely affect health and longevity. For example, increased dietary cholesterol lowers coenzyme Q-10 levels. The level is also decreased by cortisone, suggesting that stress is a factor in lowering the enzyme value.

In view of the foregoing, it is interesting to speculate that coenzyme Q-10 might play a fundamental role in decelerating aging.

PERIODONTAL DISEASE

"Your teeth are good but, your gums will have to come out" is an old joke that's all too true. Gum disease affects nine out of ten Americans in the course of a lifetime. At least one out of four people will lose all their teeth by the time they reach age sixty to gum disease. Gum disease accounts for seventy percent of all lost teeth.

More than thirty million Americans have gum disease in such an advanced state that they will lose tooth after tooth unless they get immediate dental health. Periodontal disease affects sixty percent of the young and ninety percent of all individuals over the age of sixty-five.

This doesn't have to be!

Dr. Edward G. Wilkinson, periodontal specialist and dental researcher, investigated some of the causes of gum disease while on duty with the United States Air Force. He and his co-researchers found that diseased dental tissue showed a remarkable deficiency in coenzyme Q-10. By supplementing patients with daily doses of the natural enzyme, Dr. Wilkinson and his team were able to reverse the gum conditions that were threatening the life of the teeth. Even in cases that appeared to be hopeless with no other choice but to remove the teeth to treat the gums, the use of coenzyme Q-10 showed great promise.

Proper oral hygiene and the services of a thorough dentist are helpful in every case, but healing and repair of periodontal tissue require efficient energy production.

Many studies have pointed out the deficiency of coenzyme Q-10 in gum tissue. The frequency of a deficiency ranged from 60 percent to 96 percent. Periodontitis may itself lead to a localized enzyme deficiency. However, studies have shown that 86 percent of the patients also had low levels of coenzyme Q-10 in white blood cells, indicating the presence of a systemic imbalance.

The use of supplemental coenzyme Q-10 is safe, as shown by its daily use in Japan for conditions ranging from heart disease to dental protection to life extension. As mentioned earlier, in the United States coenzyme Q-10 is available as a food supplement. The Food and Drug Administration forbids it to be advertised as anything else until its medical properties are approved.

Dr. Karl Folkers holds an FDA permit to test the substance. He has to prove it is safe and effective and, according to him, the proof is there! (Wilkinson, 1976; *also* 1977)

Clinical studies on 18 patients with periodontal disease were performed in the classic double-blind test where neither the doctors nor the patients knew which patients had received a placebo capsule and which had received a capsule containing coenzyme Q-10.

The patients took their capsules for three weeks in a row. The results were calculated according to peridontal procedure that took into account a number of factors including gingival pocket depth, swelling, bleeding, redness, pain, exudate, and looseness of teeth.

All eight patients receiving coenzyme Q-10 showed real improvement. The healing was considered to be very impressive by a group of outside dentists who had no knowledge that a test was being run. In fact, one prosthodontist remarked that the healing seen in three weeks would usually take about six months!

In an open trial, coenzyme Q-10 produced postsurgical healing that was two to three times faster than usual in seven patients suffering from advanced periodontal disease (Wilkinson, 1975). Coenzyme Q-10 may act by improving the energy-dependent processes of healing and tissue repair. It also tends to help improve abnormal citrate metabolism frequently found in many patients with periodontitis.

DIABETES MELLITUS

Diabetes is a general term for diseases characterized by excessive urination. In the form called diabetes mellitus, it is considered to be a disorder of carbohydrate metabolism characterized by hyperglycemia and glycosuria. It is the result of inadequate production or utilization of insulin.

In most instances diabetes mellitus is the result of a genetic disorder, but it may also result from a deficiency of beta cells caused by inflammation, surgery, malignancy, or other unknown problems. It is currently thought that insulin acts primarily at the cell membrane facilitating transport of glucose into the cells. Recent studies have given GTF chromium a functional role in the process.

Since it is a multifactorial illness and is associated with a number of different metabolic abnormalities, it is prudent to examine the role coenzyme Q-10 plays in this illness.

Coenzyme Q-10 is intimately involved in the metabolism of carbohydrates. Studies of diabetic rats in laboratory circumstances have shown those rats to be deficient in the enzyme. During the laboratory tests, coenzyme Q-7, which is normally present in rats as coenzyme Q-10 is normally present in humans, was administered on a supplemental basis. It was found that supplementation partly corrected abnormal glucose metabolism in alloxan-diabetic rats.

A human study of 120 diabetic patients showed that 8.3 percent were deficient in coenzyme Q-10 compared to 1.9 percent of a group of healthy people used as controls (Kishi, 1976).

When a group of diabetics using a variety of oral hypoglycemic drugs to control their diabetes were tested for coenzyme Q-10 levels, the deficiency rate was much higher. It amounted to around 20 percent, apparently because oral hypoglycemics interfere with the metabolism of the enzyme.

When the supplement was given to a group of 39 diabetics, who were in a stabilized condition, for periods ranging from two weeks to 18 weeks, the fasting blood sugar was found to be reduced by at least 20 percent in fourteen of the subjects and by at least 30 percent in twelve of the subjects (Shigeta, 1966). The dosage was 120 milligrams a day.

In some cases, when the test period was over and the supplement was withdrawn there was an increase in blood sugar or blood ketone bodies. One of the group who had difficulty controlling his condition on 60 units of insulin showed a marked fall in fasting blood sugar after supplementation.

The above studies were done with coenzyme Q-7, since coenzyme Q-10 was not available at that time. Since the Q-7 form is upgraded to Q-10, there is no reason to suspect that Q-10 will not have the same results.

We do not know how coenzyme Q-10 helps to improve diabetic control. Perhaps it induces the body to synthesize more of the enzyme itself, or perhaps it helps to enhance carbohydrate metabolism. In any event, more work is necessary to pin down the effective action, although supplementation can be done even if the mechanism is unknown.

COENZYME Q-10 AND THE CARDIOTOXICITY OF ADRIAMYCIN

Chemotherapy against malignant diseases has certain drawbacks in the way the chemotherapeutic agents interfere with normal body activities. We are all aware of the problems with falling hair, swelling, and bone and blood problems.

One particularly effective chemotherapeutic agent is called adriamycin. It has been used against certain tumors, but because it has a serious effect on the heart, particularly after treatment has gone on for some time, the use of this effective agent has been limited (Folkers, 1980).

When it was discovered that adriamycin inhibited coenzyme Q-10 dependent enzymes in tests on 11 cancer patients being treated with this drug, it was decided to use supplemental coenzyme Q-10 to see the effect (Judy, 1984). One group of seven patients received 100 milligrams of coenzyme Q-10 daily beginning three to five days before treatment with adriamycin was started. Another group of seven patients were given adriamycin but were not given any coenzyme Q-10.

The group that had received the enzyme along with the antitumor agent did not suffer the increase in cardiac problems that occurred in the group not given the supplement.

This conclusion was even more astounding since the group receiving the coenzyme Q-10 received a cumulative dosage of adriamycin about 50 percent greater than the control group. It should be noted that coenzyme Q-10 did *not* appear to protect patients with impaired cardiac function prior to adriamycin treatment.

When you take in more calories than you burn, the excess calories are stored in the form of fat. Obese people may be able to reduce the amount of stored fat by a number of methods, including reducing the intake of food, increasing the output of energy through exercise, or by increasing the efficiency of their cellular respiration and caloric output.

Certain individuals do not produce as much heat energy as others. The tendency to become overweight can, in some cases, be connected to faulty metabolic activity. Some subjects with a family history of obesity show only half the thermogenic response to food of the average person. This suggests that there is a factor in obesity that is a result of poor energy production. Since coenzyme Q-10 is an integral part of energy production on the cellular level, it is possible that a deficiency of this enzyme may play a part in some cases of obesity.

When some very obese individuals (27 subjects in all) were examined for a deficiency of coenzyme Q-10, over 50 percent or 14 of the 27 were found to be deficient (Van Gaal, 1984).

As a test, five subjects with low levels of the enzyme and a control group of four people with normal enzyme levels, were given 100 milligrams of coenzyme Q-10 daily along with a restricted diet. After nine weeks, the mean weight loss for the group that was initially deficient in coenzyme Q-10 was 13.5 kg. (a kg. is equal to 2.2 pounds) compared to a weight loss of only 5.8 kg. in the control group.

The study suggests that some individuals, perhaps up to 50 percent of really obese persons, may be deficient in coenzyme Q-10. A combination of a low-calorie diet and supplementation with the enzyme may result in a weight loss superior to that obtained by a restricted diet alone.

ATHLETIC PERFORMANCE

Another area where the concept of "bioenergetics" supplementation might enhance aerobic capacity and muscle performance is athletic performance.

A study of six healthy men not used to doing any type of exercise, sedentary in the fullest sense of the word, involved working out on a stationary bicycle (Vanfrachem, 1981). The first test was performed before taking any coenzyme Q-10 and the comparison test was done four and eight weeks after taking the supplement. The dose was 60 milligrams a day. The second test showed improved performance parameters in several areas including work capacity at submaximal heart rate, maximal oxygen consumption and oxygen transport. The improvements ranged from 3 to 12 percent.

Although much work remains to be done, the study does suggest that the use of supplementary coenzyme Q-10 could improve the physical performance of sedentary individuals.

It is also suggested that trained athletes might benefit from supplementation with improved performance and/or the relief of chronic fatigue. This possibility has yet to be investigated.

It should be printed out that most supplements on the market are in the form of 10-milligram capsules with a suggested regimen of one capsule three times a day.

COENZYME Q-10 AND THE IMMUNE SYSTEM

The immune system of the body is generally thought of as consisting of the thymus gland, the lymphatic system, the long bones of the body, the spleen, and the various products they manufacture.

Many illnesses are associated with abnormalities of the immune system. Attempts to improve the immune function of the body are standard therapy in the treatment of cancer, chronic infections, candidiasis, and acquired immune deficiency syndrome (AIDS). Just as important but seldom thought about is the energy needed by these factors to perform their jobs! Since immunity demands a constant supply of first-grade energy, coenzyme Q-10 must be in constant and adequate supply.

There have been a number of studies concerned with the immune-enhancing effect of coenzyme Q-10 in animals (Bliznakov, 1970). Studies on mice have shown that supplementation with the enzyme increased phagocytic activity of macrophages, the germ-killing ability of the white blood cells. Also, supplementation increased the number of granulocytes (other killer cells) in response to experimentally induced infection.

Coenzyme Q-10 prolonged the survival of mice which had been infected with a number of pathogenic organisms including (*Pseudomonas aeruginosa, Staphylococcus aureus, Eschericia coli, Klebsiella pneumoniae,* and *Candida albicans.* Two out of ten mice were able to survive a massive dose of *E. coli* which killed all ten of the control group.

In some human studies, eight patients with various diseases including diabetes, cancer and cardiovascular problems were given coenzyme Q-10 over a long period of time. The dosage was 60 milligrams daily (Folkers, 1982).

Significant increases in the level of immunoglobulin G (IgG) were found in the serum of these patients after three weeks to twelve weeks of supplemental treatment. This increase could represent a correction of the immunodeficiency or an increase in immunocompetence.

Immune function appears to decline with advancing age. Older mice show thymic atrophy and a marked deficiency of the enzyme. Along with that is a pronounced depression of the immune system. This depression was partially reversed when the enzyme was given on a supplemental basis, so it is possible that regular supplementation with coenzyme Q-10 may help to prevent or even to reverse age-related immunosuppression.

COENZYME Q-10 AND BETA-BLOCKERS

Prescription drugs are frequently prescribed for hypertension, and they do a marvelous job in preserving life. However, some of the drugs have side effects which, if controlled, would enable the drug to do an even better job. Propanolol and metoprolol, two of these drugs, have been found to inhibit coenzyme Q-10-dependent enzymes. It is also likely, but as yet not investigated, that many other drugs in this class have the same inhibitory effect.

In the long run, the benefits of the use from these antihypertensive agents may be compromised by the development of a coenzyme Q-10 deficiency. Therefore, supplementation with the enzyme may help to prevent a shortage of coenzyme Q-10 and may actually improve the drug's ability to help the patient.

Coenzyme Q-10 may also help to prevent other common side effects of beta-blockers, such as their reduction of cardiac contractility, or fatigue and malaise. Medical authorities should investigate the possible combination of coenzyme Q-10 and beta-blockers.

ANTIOXIDANT POWER

Free radicals occur within and without the body. The damage caused to tissues and cells by these highly reactive particles is believed to contribute to aging and to disease. Cancer, arthritis, autoimmune disease, cardiovascular disease, and other diseases are initiated or exacerbated by these free radicals.

A number of papers reveal the research done on antioxidant therapy and the way antioxidants can reduce the damaging effects of these particles. Research suggests that nutrients such as selenium, zinc, vitamin E, vitamin C, the B-complex vitamins, L-cysteine, L-methionine, and others may reduce the pathologic effects of free radicals.

Coenzyme Q-10, in addition to its role in energy production, also functions in a similar manner. In laboratory experiments, rats given the enzyme via injection had significantly fewer lipid peroxides (free radicals) in the heart and liver than a control group of animals not given the enzyme. Coenzyme Q-10 appeared to be as effective as vitamin E in the area of the heart but less effective in the liver.

The study suggests that any antioxidant program using conventional nutrients as mentioned above should also include coenzyme Q-10.

ADVERSE REACTIONS

Coenzyme Q-10 has been used for a dozen years in Japan. Millions use the enzyme on a daily basis, usually in dosages of ten milligrams, three times a day.

It is generally well tolerated and no serious adverse effects have been reported even over long-term use. It should not be used during pregnancy or lactation, not because there have been any reported problems, but simply because its safety during these periods has not yet been proven. It is contraindicated in cases of known hypersensitivity.

When a series of patients (5,143) being treated with 30 milligrams a day of coenzyme Q-10 were studied for adverse effects, the following side effects were reported:

epigastric discomfort	0.39 percent
loss of appetite	0.23 percent
nausea	0.16 percent
diarrhea	0.11 percent

This indicates the safety and tolerance this supplement offers.

Because the synthesis of new coenzyme Q-10-dependent enzymes is a slow process, response should not be expected until at least eight weeks after supplementation is started.

Bliznakov, E.G. et al. Coenzyme Q: stimulants of the phagocytic activity in rats and immune response in mice. *Experientia* 266:953, 1970.

————— et al. Coenzyme Q deficiency in aged mice. *J. Med.* 9:337, 1978.

Folkers, K. and Y. Yamura, eds. *Biomedical and Clinical Aspects of Coenzyme Q*, Vol. 2. Amsterdam: Elsevier/North Holland Biomedical Press, 1980, pp. 333-347.

Judy, W.V. et al. Coenzyme Q-10 reduction of adriamycin cardiotoxicity. In: Folkers and Yamura, Vol. 4, 1984.

Kamikawa, T. et al. Effects of coenzyme Q-10 on exercise tolerance in chronic stable angina pectoris. *Am. J. Cardiol.* 56:247, 1985.

Kishi, T. et al. Bioenergetics in clinical medicine. XI. Studies on coenzyme Q-10 and diabetes mellitus. *J. Med.* 7:307, 1976.

Mayer, P. et al. Differential effects of ubiquinone Q-7 and ubiquinone analogs on macrophage activation and experimental infections in granulocytopenic mice. *Infection* 8:256, 1980.

Oda, T. and K. Hamamoto. Effect of coenzyme Q-10 on the stress-induced decrease of cardiac performance in pediatric patients with mitral valve prolapse. *Jpn. Circ. J.* 48:1387, 1984.

Shigeta, Y. et al. Effect of coenzyme Q-7 treatment on blood sugar and ketone bodies of diabetics. *J. Vitaminol.* 12:293, 1966.

Suzuki, H. et al. Cardiac performance and coenzyme Q-10 in thyroid disorders. *Endocrinol. Japan.* 31:755, 1984.

Vanfrachem, J. H. P. and K. Folkers. *Coenzyme Q-10 and Clinical Aspects of Coenzyme 9.* Amsterdam: Biomedical Press, 1981.

Van Gaal, L. et al. Exploratory study of coenzyme Q-10 in obesity. In: Folkers and Yamura, Vol. 4, 1984, pp 369-373.

Wilkinson, E. G. et al. Bioenergetics in clinical medicine. II. Adjunctive treatment with coenzyme Q in periodontal therapy. *Res. Commun. Chem. Pathol. Pharmacol.* 12:111, 1975.

————— et al. Bioenergetics in clinical medicine. VI. Adjunctive treatment with coenzyme Q in periodontal therapy. *Res. Commun. Chem. Pathol, Pharmacol.* 14:715, 1976.

————— et al. Treatment of periodontal and other soft tissue diseases of the oral cavity with coenzyme Q. In: Folkers and Yamura, Vol. 1, 1977, pp 251-265.

Yamagami, T. et al. Reduction by coenzyme Q-10 of hypertension induced by deoxycorticosterone and saline in rats. *Internat. J. Vit. Nutr. Res.* 44:487, 1974.

————— et al. Correlation between serum coenzyme Q levels and succinate dehydrogenase coenzyme Q reductase activity in cardiovascular disease and the influence of coenzyme Q administration. In: Folkers and Yamura, Vol. 1, 1977, pp 251-265.